Mind Diet Cookbook

50 Memory Boosting Meals

Reduce The Risk Of Developing Alzheimer's Disease

By: Gabrielle Sanders

Table Of Contents

Introduction

Boost your brain health and reduce your risks of developing Alzheimer's disease by eating delicious, nutritious, and easy-to-make meals.

If you're reading this book, chances are you've seen for yourself what Alzheimer's disease can do to a person. Today, there are approximately 27 million people all over the globe who are suffering from Alzheimer's disease. In fact, it is the sixth leading cause of mortality in the United States. The worst thing about this disease is that it is progressive and irreversible. Not only does it take away your future but it also robs you of your past. It's for this reason why focusing on prevention is extremely important. Through the decades, people have been formulating meal plans for weight loss, diets to improve athletic performance, and even recipes for better looking skin. It's high time that we concentrate on a fitness program that's focused on improving not just the body but the mind as well.

Research reveals that there are certain foods that can help boost brain performance and sharpen the memory. These include foods that are rich in complex B vitamins, antioxidants, and unsaturated fatty acids. The MIND diet is all about incorporating these power foods into your daily meals so that you get to reap the holistic health benefits. We're talking about wellness from top to bottom.

Through this book, you'll learn more about the MIND diet and how it can help you in building your best line of defense against the development of Alzheimer's disease and dementia. You'll also find 50 of the best MIND diet recipes for breakfast, lunch, dinner, and even for those moments in between. The greatest thing about these recipes is that they don't require any hard-to-find or expensive ingredients. Read on to feed your brain with knowledge and afterwards, head to the kitchen and feed your body and your mind with these healthy and flavorsome meals.

Thanks again for buying this book, I hope you enjoy it!

Chapter 1

Eating from the Top Down

What You Need to Know About Alzheimer's

Alzheimer's is a brain disease which creates problems with the affected person's memory, thinking, and how he behaves. It is important to emphasize that the memory loss and changes in behavior associated with Alzheimer's are not a normal part of the aging process. The disease inevitably worsens overtime. Among the first noticeable symptoms of Alzheimer's disease is extreme forgetfulness which is enough to lessen the person's overall quality of life. It's the kind of forgetfulness that dramatically decreases work productivity, affects one's personal relationships, and even takes away one's ability to enjoy activities which he used to love. That said, Alzheimer's disease begins by corrupting the brain at a microscopic level long before any signs of the disease becomes noticeable.

Our brain consists of a hundred billion neurons. Each nerve cell links to several other nerve cells to establish a network of communication. Additionally, the brain also has cells which work to provide support and nourishment to the other brain cells. Think of your brain as a huge factory where each cell has an important job to perform. Some are for thinking. Some are for learning. Some are for remembering. Some are for smelling, hearing, seeing, or instructing the muscles how and when to move. To keep the entire brain factory running, coordination, nutrition, and adequate oxygenation are all equally essential. Though the exact cause and mechanism of Alzheimer's is still unknown, experts believe that the disease begins when one of the "workers" in the factory malfunctions. One of the neurons breaks down and gradually takes the entire factory down with it.

All that is known at present is that the brains of patients who are suffering from Alzheimer's disease contain more developed plaques and tangles compared to the brains of normal healthy elderly individuals. Plaques are protein deposits which form in the areas between the neurons. Meanwhile, tangles are gnarled protein fibers which form within the nerve cells. Furthermore, the plaques and tangles in persons with Alzheimer's disease tend to develop in a foreseeable pattern. They start from the parts of the brain which are essential for memory prior to spreading to other areas. The current strongest theory is that these plaques and tangles work to hinder communication between the nerve cells and thus, interrupt the normal processes required by the cells in order to survive.

Research reveals that individuals who are most at risk for developing Alzheimer's disease are elderly folks aged 65 and above and persons with a family history of Alzheimer's. That said, studies also show that there are foods which actually increase one's predisposition for developing Alzheimer's and dementia. As previously mentioned, your brain requires a healthy combination of oxygen and nutrients in order for the cells to remain in top condition. When you consume less foods which contain essential vitamins, minerals, and healthy fats while eating more complex carbs, sugar, and processed food items, this triggers the creation of inflammatory toxins. This leads to the formation of plaques in the brain which as formerly stated, impairs one's cognitive functions. Thankfully, there are also foods which can help nourish the brain cells and thus, support cerebral function.

What is the MIND diet and how can it help you prevent the onset of Alzheimer's disease and dementia?

MIND is an acronym which means:

Mediterranean-DASH

Intervention for

Neurodegenerative

Delay.

In other words, it's a mash up between the popular Mediterranean diet and the heart-friendly DASH diet and combines all of the goodness from both meal plans. In the Mediterranean fitness plan, the dieters consume plenty of fruits and veggies, healthy grains and beans and nuts, fish oils, and olive oil while keeping the intake of meat and dairy to a minimum. Furthermore, the Mediterranean lifestyle promotes daily exercise and sharing hearty meals with good company preferably with some fine red wine. Meanwhile, the DASH diet is a dietary approach geared towards stopping hypertension dead in its tracks. Like the Mediterranean diet, the DASH diet encourages followers to eat more fruits and veggies. Dieters are also asked to consume low-fat dairy while cutting back on cholesterol-rich food sources and foods that contain high amounts of saturated fat and trans fats. The consumption of whole grains, poultry, and fish are also encouraged. All the while, you'll need to limit your intake of sweets, salts, and red meat. As you may have noticed, both diets are extremely beneficial for the body.

So what makes the MIND diet different?

The main difference between the MIND diet and the two other diets mentioned is that the former specifically encourages the consumption of foods and nutrients which are scientifically known to be beneficial for the brain. You include brain-boosting ingredients in your recipes while implementing a low-salt, low-sugar, low-cholesterol diet with lots of fresh fruits and vegetables and organic meats.

What foods are you allowed to eat?

When following the MIND diet, always make sure that each meal consists mostly of any of the following food groups:

- **Green leafy veggies** such as spinach, lettuce, Brussels sprouts, arugula, collard greens, and kale

  Make sure that you have a minimum of six servings per week.

- A healthy assortment of non-leafy **vegetables** like squash, beets, tomatoes, peas, endives, zucchini, and eggplant at least once daily

  According to nutrition experts, in order for your daily diet plan to be highly beneficial for the brain, it should consist of one salad meal and one other vegetable.

- **Nuts** such as almonds, walnuts, cashews, and pistachios

  Instead of grabbing a sugary snack in between meals, munch on these filling brain foods instead. Nuts are rich in fats which makes them satisfying so you'll end up losing your craving for carbs. They are also high in antioxidants and fiber. More than that, studies show that regular consumption of nuts lead to a reduction of bad cholesterol in the body, thus lowering one's risk of developing heart disease.

According to the MIND diet plan, you should have five servings of nuts per week.

- **Berries** like blueberries, raspberries, and strawberries are powerful brain-boosting fruits which helps improve one's cognitive function. It's advised that you take ½ cup of fresh berries at least two times per week.

- **Beans** should be included in the diet at least thrice per week. You can do this by consuming ½ cup of beans every other day.

- Meanwhile, **whole grains** like buckwheat, faro, barley, oats, and quinoa should be taken more frequently. Include three or more servings in your daily meal plan.

- Omega 3 fatty acids in **wild-caught fish** like salmon, tuna, trout, and halibut are not just beneficial for the heart but for the brain as well. While the Mediterranean diet suggests that you eat fish almost every other day, the MIND diet recommends having them at least once a week only.

- Chicken lovers will be glad to know that **poultry** is a part of this brain-boosting nutrition plan. You are advised to eat organic poultry such as chicken, turkey, geese, and duck at least two times per week.

- When cooking, the MIND diet strongly recommends that you use **olive oil**. Compared to other oils used for cooking, olive oil consists of more healthy fats thus contributing to satiety. Studies show that individuals and families who frequently use olive oil at home are less likely to suffer from cognitive decline.
- The MIND diet also advises the consumption of *one* glass of red wine to go with a healthy meal. Wine is to be taken optionally and once a day only.

What foods should you avoid?

While **red meat** should not be eliminated entirely, you should minimize its consumption to less than four servings per week. That's if you want to preserve your brain health. When it comes to red meats, the MIND diet cuts you a bit more slack than the Mediterranean diet which limits red meat consumption to one serving per week only.

When possible, olive oil should take the place of **butter and margarine**. When necessary for a recipe, limit the use of butter or margarine to one tablespoonful per day.

To reduce the odds of you and your family developing Alzheimer's in the future, cut down **cheese** consumption to a maximum of one serving each week.

Sweet treats and pastries are not completely prohibited but you'll need to limit intake to five servings weekly or even less.

Eating of **fried food** should be reduced to one serving per week.

Fast food is generally not encouraged but if you can't avoid them, then at least refrain from eating fast food more than once a week.

What are the other benefits of the MIND diet?

Apart from lowering your risk of developing Alzheimer's and dementia by as much as 54%, the MIND diet brings in plenty of other benefits like normalized cholesterol levels, reduced risk for obesity, and better overall health. Because the MIND diet limits the consumption of unhealthy foods which lead to weight gain, you're not just helping your brain cells but your waistline as well.

Another great thing about the MIND diet is that it's not as strict as the Mediterranean diet, the DASH diet, or any other popular diets out there. Because of this, you're more likely to adhere faithfully to the meal plan in the long run. Furthermore, studies show that even *part-time* followers of the MIND diet are still less likely to develop Alzheimer's by 35%! Meanwhile, hardcore followers of the Mediterranean diet *only* or the DASH diet *only* reflect no drop in Alzheimer's risk at all.

The MIND diet is convenient and does not demand the use of pricey, impossible-to-find ingredients. All ingredients are easily attainable and reasonably affordable. Since moderate consumption of alcohol is allowed, this diet plan is a whole lot more realistic and achievable. This is important because a lot of the time, when people are unable to stick to their strict diet goals, they end up in a nasty downward spiral back towards their unhealthy "comfort foods".

You know how sometimes you just want to eat breakfast for dinner? In the MIND diet, there are no strict and specific breakfast, lunch, or dinner suggestions. In other words, you can eat whatever you want whenever you want to as long as it's within the recommended food group and within the suggested frequency. So if you want to eat berries and nuts for dinner or an arugula and tuna salad for breakfast, it's okay. This way, you can pair the heaviness of your meal with the type of activities you have scheduled during the day.

Dining out is not a problem with the MIND diet either. As long as you minimize your visits to greasy fast food chains, skip the entrees slathered with cheese and butter, and pass on the sugar-filled dessert, you'll still be able to have a social life!

The MIND diet does not involve rigorous calorie counting. Because there are no calorie-cutting requirements in the MIND diet, you are free to feel as full as you want with fiber-rich leafy greens. This is important because when you reach the level of satiety from healthy food sources, you'll crave unhealthy foods less and less.

Chapter 2

Brain-boosting Broths

Carrot Soup for Cognitive Health

Ingredients:

- 450 g carrots
- 4 oz. plain yogurt
- 24 oz. vegetable broth
- 2 tbsp. olive oil
- 8 oz. onion, yellow variety
- ½ tsp. cinnamon, ground
- 1 ½ tsp. cumin, ground
- 1 tsp. turmeric, ground
- 1 tsp. fresh lemon juice
- desired amount of salt and pepper (minimize salt)
- raw wild honey to sweeten

Directions:

1. Chop the onions. Peel and dice the carrots to ½ inch cubes.

2. Adjust the stove's setting to medium high. In a large saucepan, heat the olive oil. Sauté the chopped yellow onions for a couple of minutes then throw in the carrots. Keep sautéing just until the onions are partly brown and soft.

3. Pour in the vegetable broth. Add the spices.

4. Allow to boil.

5. Once the soup starts boiling, lower the heat and replace the lid on the saucepan.

6. Leave to simmer until the carrots are softened. This should take approximately less than half an hour.

7. Afterwards, remove the saucepan from heat. Leave to cool.

8. Then, use a blender to puree the mixture until it's nice and smooth.

9. Next, pour the smooth mixture back into the saucepan. Over low heat, add desired amount of honey and the teaspoonful of lemon juice.

10. Sprinkle desired amount of salt and pepper.

11. Serve this memory boosting soup with a drizzle of plain yogurt.

Note: Carrots are rich in beta carotene which has potent antioxidant properties. Studies reveal that individuals with beta carotene deficiency commonly suffer from cognitive decline as they age. Apart from providing you with a healthy dose of beta carotene, this recipe enables you to benefit from memory boosting spices like cinnamon, onions, and turmeric.

Winter-perfect Turkey and Kale Soup

Ingredients:

- 250 g turkey
- 40 oz. chicken stock, organic
- 32 oz. kale
- 3 medium-sized carrots, shaved
- 12 oz. cauliflower, minced
- 15 oz. fresh tomatoes
- 2 tbsp. olive oil
- 4 shallots
- 1 bell pepper
- minimal amount of sea salt (a pinch will do)
- black pepper, freshly ground

Directions:

1. Chop the shallots. Dice the carrots and slice the bell pepper. Cut the tomatoes into chunks. Remove the ribs from the kale and chop up the leaves.
2. Adjust the stove's setting to medium high. In a saucepan, add the olive oil and heat it up.
3. Then, throw in the chopped shallots, cauliflowers, carrots, and bell pepper.

4. Sauté the veggies for about nine minutes or until they are almost tender.
5. Next, add the turkey meat and cook for approximately 7 minutes.
6. Pour in the chicken broth. This is to be followed by the tomatoes.
7. Sprinkle desired amount of salt and pepper.
8. Allow the soup to boil.
9. When it starts to boil, add the kale. Adjust the stove's setting to low and tend to the soup with continuous stirring.
10. Afterwards, replace the lid of the saucepan and leave to simmer for about 13-16 minutes.
11. Enjoy!

Brain Buddy Blueberry Soup

Ingredients:

- 680 g blueberries, fresh
- 4 oz. pineapple juice, freshly squeezed from a juicer
- 20 oz. water
- 3 tbsp. Chambord liquor
- 1 tsp. vanilla essence
- juice from 1 lime
- 2 tsp. orange peel
- a pinch of natural salt

Directions:

1. In a small-sized saucepan, boil the Chambord liquor until it is reduced down to half. Leave to cool.
2. Next, pour the cooled liquor into a blender. Throw in the rest of the ingredients.
3. Process until the mixture is pureed smoothly.
4. Use a strainer to purify 50% of the mixture. Then, pour the strained soup back with the unstrained half.

5. Mix thoroughly and enjoy with lively company.

Barley and Veggie Soup

Ingredients:

- 32 g. dry barley
- 32 oz. water
- 1 tbsp. olive oil
- 2 oz. carrots, diced
- ½ tsp. garlic, finely chopped
- 2 oz. onions, yellow variety, diced
- 9 oz. button mushrooms, sliced
- 2 oz. green peas
- 2 tbsp. tamari sauce (choose the low sodium variety)
- 2 oz. potatoes, diced
- 1 tsp. natural sea salt
- black pepper, freshly ground

Directions:

1. After rinsing the barley, place it in a big saucepan.
2. Pour in the water. Then, leave it to boil.
3. Once the water boils, adjust the stove's setting to low. Replace the lid of the saucepan and allow to simmer for about 22 minutes.
4. Add the low-sodium tamari. Stir well.
5. Obtain a smaller pan and adjust the stove's setting to medium.

6. Add the olive oil and sauté the garlic and the onions until the latter is soft.
7. Throw in the mushrooms and sauté until they're tender. Then, transfer the sautéed ingredients into the bigger saucepan with the soup.
8. Next, it's time to add the potatoes and the carrots into the broth. Replace the lid of the saucepan and simmer for about 23 minutes. The potatoes should be soft by then.
9. Finally, turn off the heat and add the peas.
10. Season with salt and pepper.
11. Serve while still hot.

Special Salmon Chowder

Ingredients:

- 1 ½ lbs. wild salmon fillets
- 28 oz. tomatoes, crushed
- 16 oz. vegetable broth
- 2 oz. olive oil
- 4 oz. celery, chopped
- 4 oz. onion, chopped
- 4 oz. carrots, chopped
- ½ tsp. thyme
- 1 pc. bay leaf
- desired amount of sea salt and black pepper

Directions:

1. Cut the salmon fillet into cubes that are about ¾ inch in size. Ensure that all of the bones are removed. If you prefer, you can also peel off the skin with the edge of a sharp knife. Alternatively, you can ask the fish vendor to do this for you. Rub with salt and pepper.

2. Adjust the stove's setting to medium. Heat the olive oil in a large pot with a heavy bottom.

3. Next, throw in the carrots, the celery, and the onion. Sauté for approximately 5 minutes.

4. After that, pour in the vegetable broth. Add the tomatoes. Follow this up with the bay leaf and the thyme.

5. Replace the lid of the pot and allow to simmer for about 15 minutes.

6. After this, it's time to add the salmon. Cook for another 12-16 minutes with occasional stirring.

7. Then, take the bay leaf out.

8. Season with fresh herbs like some tarragon or more thyme.

9. Serve.

Memory Broth

Ingredients:

- 256 oz. water
- 3 medium-sized carrots
- 2 onions, white variety
- 1 parsnip
- a couple of stalks of celery
- a couple of bulbs of fennel
- 2 oz. ginger, peeled and sliced
- a bunch of scallions
- half a bundle of flat-leaf parsley stems
- a stem of lemongrass
- 1 tsp. dehydrated oregano
- 1 tsp. dehydrated rosemary
- 2 fresh cloves
- 1 pc. bay leaf
- 1 tsp. black peppercorns
- 1 tsp. powdered turmeric
- 1 tsp. sea salt

Directions:

1. Slice the carrots. Cut the lemongrass stalk to half lengthways. Chop the onions, the garlic, celery, the parsnip, and the fennel.
2. In a big-sized pot, mix all of the ingredients together.

3. Adjust the stove's setting to high and leave to boil.
4. When the soup is boiling, reduce the heat, remove the lid from the pot, and allow the broth so simmer for a couple of hours.
5. Afterwards, use a fine-mesh strainer to strain the soup.
6. Serve immediately.

Note: Because you'll be making a potful of broth with these proportions, you can keep the rest in the fridge for future consumption. The average shelf life of this recipe is 2 weeks.

Warming Red Lentil Soup

Ingredients:

- 48 oz. vegetable stock
- 8 oz. red lentils
- 2 oz. onions
- 2 oz. carrots
- ¼ tsp. dehydrated basil
- 2 oz. celery
- 1 tbsp. garlic, finely chopped
- ½ tsp. Worcestershire sauce
- 1 tbsp. olive oil, extra virgin
- a pinch of dehydrated thyme
- a pinch of dehydrated oregano
- 1 ½ tsp. white vinegar, distilled
- 1 tsp. sea salt
- ¼ tsp. black pepper, freshly ground

Directions:

1. Chop the onions, the celery, and the carrots.
2. Adjust the stove's setting to medium heat and prepare a big saucepan.
3. Add the olive oil to be heated.
4. Cook the carrots along with the garlic, the celery, and the onions until the latter is transparent.
5. Pour in the vegetable stock.

6. Next, throw in the lentils and the dried herbs. Leave to boil.
7. Once the soup is boiling, adjust the stove's setting to low.
8. Leave to simmer for 60 minutes with the saucepan's lid on.
9. After that, turn off the stove and allow the soup to cool down.
10. Then, transfer the mixture into a blender. Process until you are able to get a smooth puree.
11. Add the rest of the ingredients for flavor with thorough stirring.
12. Share the warmth with friends and family!

Powerful Carrot and Turmeric Brew

Ingredients:

- 48 oz. carrots, peeled and chopped
- 2 tbsp. fresh turmeric root, grated
- 32 oz. vegetable broth
- 1 small-sized onion, white variety, diced
- ¼ tsp. powdered cinnamon
- 2 garlic cloves, finely chopped
- 1 tbsp. fresh ginger, grated
- a dash of red pepper bits
- 1 tbsp. olive oil
- ½ tsp. sea salt
- 4 oz. coconut milk

Directions:

1. Start by heating the olive oil in a big, heavy bottomed pot. Adjust the stove's setting to medium high. Sauté the onions for about 6 minutes until translucent. Be sure to introduce a few tablespoonsful of water while doing this so the onions won't stick.
2. Next, add the ginger, the garlic, and the turmeric and sauté for another couple of minutes until the fragrant aroma is released.

3. Then, pour in the vegetable broth.
4. Add the carrots. Follow this up with the pepper bits and the cinnamon.
5. Sprinkle the salt.
6. Leave the soup to boil.
7. Once it's boiling, adjust the stove's setting to low.
8. Replace the lid of the pot and leave to simmer for about half an hour.
9. Once done, pour the mixture into an immersion blender. You may have to divide it into a few batches. Process until the mixture is smooth.
10. If you think the soup is a bit too thick for your taste, feel free to add 4-6 oz. more vegetable broth.
11. The next thing you should do is to add the coconut milk. Stir well and taste. If you like, you can top the dish with turmeric powder.
12. This recipe is good for five people so feel free to share this meal with loved ones!

Note: When stored in the fridge inside an airtight container, this soup can last for more than three days. When kept in the freezer, it can last for as long as 4 weeks.

This recipe is also best served with some roasted chickpeas. For the recipe, check out the next chapter.

Chapter 3

Mini Meals for Your Memory

Flavorful Toasted Chickpeas

Ingredients:

- 16 oz. chickpeas, cooked
- 1 tsp. ground cumin
- 1 tsp. chili powder
- 1 tbsp. olive oil
- ¼ tsp. paprika
- sea salt
- freshly ground black pepper

Directions:

1. Heat up the oven to 400 F. Prior to roasting the chickpeas, toss them in the olive oil. Coat them with the chili, then with the cumin, and then with the paprika.
2. Arrange the chickpeas evenly into a baking pan lined with parchment.
3. Sprinkle with desired amount of pepper and just a little bit of natural sea salt.

4. Roasting time is between 33 to 37 minutes. The chickpeas should be crispy and they should yield a beautiful golden brown hue.

5. Be sure to stir the peas from time to time so they won't end up sticking.

6. Serve alone as a snack or for breakfast. Alternatively, you can serve ¾ cup of this recipe along with the Powerful Carrot and Turmeric Brew for a full meal on a busy day.

Note: When kept in an airtight container, this recipe can have a shelf life of up to 7 days.

Gallo Pinto from Costa Rica

Ingredients:

- 4 oz. black beans
- a cup of rice, cooked
- ¼ tsp. cumin
- 1 small-sized clove of garlic, finely chopped
- 1 tsp. olive oil
- 4 oz. water
- 1 tsp. vinegar, organic
- a squeeze of lime juice
- sea salt
- freshly ground black pepper

Directions:

1. Adjust the stove's setting to medium heat.
2. Pour the water into a saucepan. Then, add the beans. Cook for a couple of minutes.
3. Next, pour in the olive oil and the vinegar. Throw in the cumin, the pepper, and the garlic. Cook for another three minutes.

4. Then, lower the heat. Introduce the rice to the water. Heat the rice until it ends up very warm. That said, refrain from boiling the rice.

5. Squeeze some lime juice over the mixture.

6. Use a tiny bit of salt and some more pepper for seasoning.

7. Top with chopped cilantro if you like. Cilantro is also a known memory-boosting ingredient.

8. Enjoy your meal!

Note: To make this meal more filling, you can top it with slices of avocado. You can also dice some precooked vegetables and add them to your meal. Zucchini tastes great with this recipe.

Easy Rice and Barley Recipe

Ingredients:

- 28 g pearled barley, quick cook variety
- 85 g rice, precooked
- 2 tbsp. vinegar
- Himalayan sea salt to taste

Directions:

1. Rinse the barley several times. Then, place it in a small-sized saucepan.
2. Add 9 oz. water.
3. Afterwards, pour in the vinegar.
4. Stir well.
5. Adjust the stove's setting to medium heat. Cook the barley for about 11 minutes.
6. Next, add the precooked rice. Cook for another 60 seconds.
7. Then, replace the lid of the saucepan and turn off the heat. Leave for about two and a half minutes.
8. Add a bit of salt for seasoning.

Extreme Egg Congee

Ingredients:

- 85 g rice, precooked
- oz. water
- 1 tsp. olive oil
- 1 big egg, organic
- 1 tsp. vinegar

Directions:

1. Beat the egg.
2. Adjust the stove's setting to medium heat.
3. In a medium-sized saucepan, pour in the water.
4. Then, add the rice and the egg. Stir.
5. Add the teaspoonful of olive oil followed by the vinegar. Mix well.
6. Afterwards, adjust the stove's setting to low. Replace the lid of the saucepan and cook for 9-11 minutes with occasional stirring.
7. For a thicker porridge, simply use less water. For a thinner porridge, just add more water.

8. Season with black pepper and a tiny bit of salt.

Note: If you're in a rush, you can shorten the cooking time of the porridge by crushing the rice with a fork beforehand.

You can turn this recipe into a savory meal or a sweet meal. For a sweet porridge, just use a few slices or apples, apricot, or peach or some blueberries as toppings. Increase the nutritional value of this dish by sprinkling some nuts on top too. Walnuts and pecans taste fantastic with this recipe.

Classic Greek Salad

Ingredients:

- 16 oz. lettuce
- 1 big plum tomato
- half of a big-sized cucumber
- 3 oz. feta cheese, crumbled
- 5 slices of onion, red
- 2 oz. black olives
- ½ green pepper
- ½ red pepper

Directions:

1. Shred the lettuce leaves. Peel and slice the cucumber. Chop the red and green peppers and then the olives.
2. Get a bowl and fill it with some ice water. Soak the onions for 8-12 minutes. This will help lessen the intensity of the taste. Afterwards, dry the onion rings. Slice them up.
3. Arrange all of the ingredients save for the feta cheese in a salad bowl.
4. Add the dressing. (see next recipe) Toss well.

5. Arrange the feta cheese on top of the salad.

Note: This recipe is good for two so feel free to share it with someone whose company you enjoy!

Classic Greek Salad Dressing

Note: This dressing recipe is not just for the salad recipe mentioned above. This works great with just about any assortment of green leafy veggies and fruit combos that are meant to be eaten raw. The proportions in this recipe are good for 4 servings.

Ingredients:

- 3 oz. olive oil, extra virgin
- 1 ½ tbsp. lemon juice
- 1 ½ tbsp. vinegar, organic
- 1 clove garlic, minced
- freshly ground black pepper
- 1 tsp. oregano
- ½ tsp. sea salt

Directions:

1. Combine all of the ingredients in a food processor.

2. Pour over your salad and enjoy!

Japanese Style Ginger Salad

Ingredients:

- 2 oz. olive oil
- 2 tbsp. organic apple cider vinegar
- 2 tbsp. low-sodium soy sauce
- 2 tbsp. celery, minced
- 1 tbsp. fresh gingerroot, minced
- 2 tbsp. spring onion, minced
- 1 tsp. fresh lime juice
- freshly ground black pepper

Directions:

1. Combine all of the ingredients in a food processor.
2. Process well and pour over a balanced mix of raw greens and other veggies.
3. The proportions in this recipe are good for 6 servings.

Tasty Chickpea and Lima Bean Tapenade

Ingredients:

- 15 oz. lima beans
- 8 medium-sized olives
- 1 tbsp. organic apple cider vinegar
- 1 tbsp. parsley
- 2 tsp. lemon juice
- 15 oz. garbanzos
- 8 oz. water
- 1 clove of garlic
- 1 fresh mint
- ¼ red pepper bits, crushed
- 1 tbsp. olive oil, extra virgin
- 1 tbsp. fresh parsley
- 1 tsp. capers
- black pepper, freshly ground
- natural sea salt

Directions:

1. Drain the beans. Chop up the capers and the olives. Press the clove of garlic. Mince the mint and the parsley.

2. Pour the water in a saucepan. Add the lima beans and the garbanzos and cook for about 9-12 minutes.

3. Afterwards, place the beans in a medium-sized bowl. Use a fork to mash them up so you could make bean paste. Alternatively, you can throw them together in a food processor.

4. Add the rest of the ingredients into the bowl. Mix well.

5. Slather this on top of raw veggies, toast, or crackers.

6. This recipe serves 5 persons so feel free to share with guests!

Couscous Salad Provencal

The proportions in this recipe are enough to provide a light meal for 7 persons.

Ingredients:

- 85 g couscous, uncooked
- 3 medium-sized tomatoes
- 16 oz. parsley, finely chopped
- 1 tsp. sea salt
- 10 oz. water
- 2 tbsp. olive oil, extra virgin
- 24 oz. mint, finely chopped
- 2 oz. fresh lemon juice
- 2 tbsp. white wine vinegar
- a few grinds of fresh black pepper

Directions:

1. Start by chopping up the tomatoes. Then, put them in a colander by the sink.
2. Throw in half a teaspoonful of sea salt. Mix thoroughly and allow to drain for half an hour.

3. In a big bowl, place the couscous. Add the couple of tablespoonsful of olive oil and make sure that you spread it evenly.
4. Meanwhile, get the water boiling. Afterwards, add the couscous.
5. Use a fork for fluffing the couscous.
6. Cook for about 14-16 minutes.
7. After that, add the lemon juice and the white wine vinegar.
8. Follow this up with the parsley, the mint, and the rest of the salt.
9. Lastly, add the pepper and the tomatoes. Mix well.

Brain-boosting Breakfast Scramble

Ingredients:

- 2 big eggs, organic
- 32 g black beans, cooked
- half of a small-sized avocado, diced
- 2 tsp. olive oil
- 2 oz. onion
- 1 garlic clove, finely chopped
- 4 oz. white bottom mushrooms
- 2 grinds of fresh black pepper
- cilantro leaves (optional)
- 1/8 tsp. salt, preferably kosher

Directions:

1. First, cook the mushrooms and the onions in olive oil for approximately 5 minutes. When the onions are tender, throw in the garlic and sauté for an extra 60 seconds.
2. Break the eggs into a bowl. Whisk. Then, pour the beaten eggs over the garlic, the onions, and the mushrooms.

3. Next, add the precooked black beans.
4. Sprinkle with some salt and pepper.
5. Cook the eggs with constant stirring.
6. Transfer to a plate. Use the avocado and the cilantro as toppings.

The Ultimate Kale and Blueberry Salad

Ingredients:

- 3 bunches of kale
- 4.5 oz. blueberries
- 2 carrots, julienned
- 1 tbsp. mint leaves, chopped
- 2.25 oz. pomegranate seeds
- 4 oz. soy sesame vinaigrette (recipe to follow)
- 1/5 oz. almonds, toasted and sliced
- 1.5 oz. toasted pumpkin seeds
- kosher salt
- black pepper, freshly ground

Directions:

1. Wash the kale, remove the stems, and chop up the leaves coarsely.
2. Place the leafy greens in a medium-sized salad bowl.
3. Add the seeds, the blueberries, and the carrots. Mix.

4. Throw in the almonds and the mint. Toss.
5. Toss again after drizzling with the soy sesame vinaigrette.
6. Add salt and pepper for seasoning.
7. Dig in!

Soy Sesame Vinaigrette Recipe

Ingredients:

- 8 oz. rice vinegar
- 2 oz. sesame oil
- 4 oz. low-sodium soy sauce
- 2 tbsp. cornstarch
- 2 oz. peanut oil
- 4 oz. mirin
- 3.88 oz. brown sugar
- a pinch of red pepper bits
- 2 tbsp. fresh ginger, minced
- 2 tbsp. garlic, chopped
- 2 tbsp. water

Directions:

1. In a blender, mix the peanut and sesame oils. Then, throw in the garlic, the pepper bits, and the ginger. Process together until you get a nice and creamy puree.
2. Adjust the stove's setting to low heat. Pour the oil blend into a medium-sized saucepan. Cook with continuous stirring

until it turns golden brown. This should take about five minutes or slightly longer.

3. Afterwards, pour in the soy sauce, the vinegar, and the mirin. Add the sugar as well.

4. Mix the water and the cornstarch in a bowl.

5. Then, pour the mixture into the saucepan.

6. Bring the sauce to a boil while maintaining the low heat setting. Allow the sauce to thicken with continuous stirring. This should take about a couple of minutes.

7. After this, you can pour the vinaigrette into a bowl and leave it there to cool. Pour over your kale and blueberry salad or any green leafy veggie and fruit combo.

Note: When kept in the fridge, this vinaigrette has a shelf life of about 7 days.

Banana-Avocado Smoothie

Ingredients:

- a large-sized avocado
- a big banana
- 4 oz. yogurt
- 2 tbsp. raw wild honey
- 6 pcs. ice cubes

Directions:

1. Combine all of the ingredients together in a blender.
2. Process until you get a smooth texture.
3. Drink up for a quick and healthy mind-boosting snack or breakfast.

Why avocadoes? It's true that avocados have earned a negative rep for their rich fat content. Nevertheless, when taken in moderate amounts, they are very potent brain foods. Being rich in monounsaturated fats, avocadoes can actually help decrease blood pressure and boost blood flow. These two factors greatly contribute to a dramatic decrease of cognitive deterioration.

Type 2 diabetes is a known risk factor for Alzheimer's disease. That said, the monounsaturated fats in avocadoes inhibits insulin resistance. Also, the polyphenols and flavonoids found in avocadoes perform anti-inflammatory functions which help combat Alzheimer's. Meanwhile, the vitamin K found in this fruit also helps promote blood circulation. Moreover, avocadoes are also rich in folate so they can help hinder the development of protein tangles associated with Alzheimer's. Avocadoes are also a good source of omega 3 fatty acids.

Healthy Avocado and White Bean Salad

Ingredients:

- 14 oz. white beans
- 1 ½ tbsp. olive oil
- 1 avocado
- 1 Roma tomato
- 2 oz. lemon juice
- dehydrated basil
- garlic powder
- sea salt
- 1 tsp. mustard
- black pepper, freshly ground

Directions:

1. Chop up the avocado and the tomato.
2. In a bowl, mix the lemon juice, the olive oil, and the mustard.
3. Add the salt, pepper, basil, and garlic powder.
4. Sprinkle salt and pepper.
5. Whisk well.
6. Arrange the white beans, the tomato cubes and the avocado slices in a bowl.
7. Pour the vinaigrette over the salad.

8. Mix.
9. Place in the fridge and serve cold.

Tuna Lettuce Wraps with Avocado

Ingredients:

- 3 oz. tuna flakes, boiled
- ½ avocado, ripe
- 2 big lettuce leaves
- 2 oz. green olives, cut into halves
- 2 tbsp. green chilies, diced
- 1 spring onion, diced

Directions:

1. Use a fork to mash the avocado in a small bowl.
2. Next, add the tuna, the olives, the chilies, and the spring onion.
3. Scoop the tuna mixture into each lettuce leaf.
4. Bon apetit!

Quinoa Sushi Rolls

Ingredients:

- 85 g quinoa
- 4 pcs. nori sheets
- 1 large avocado
- 1 small-sized cucumber, organic
- 16 oz. water
- 3 tbsp. brown rice vinegar
- a fistful of spinach
- 1 tsp. raw wild honey
- a pinch of sea salt

Directions:

1. In a saucepan, pour in the water and add the quinoa. Bring to a boil.
2. Once boiling, lower the heat and leave to simmer until the quinoa is fully cooked.
3. Slice the cucumber and the avocado thinly.
4. In a small bowl, combine the brown rice vinegar, the honey, and the salt.
5. Slowly pour the mixture over the quinoa with continuous mixing.
6. Slather the quinoa all over each sushi wrap. Make sure that you leave a couple of inches at the edge of the wrap.

7. Put some spinach on top of the quinoa. Then, add the cucumber and avocado slices on top of the spinach.
8. Roll each wrap snugly and slice them up.
9. Serve.

Blueberry-Avocado Brain Power Smoothie

Ingredients:

- a handful of blueberries
- 1 medium-sized avocadoes, ripe
- 1 big banana
- a dash of chia seeds
- a couple of oz. of pomegranate juice
- 6 pcs. ice cubes

Directions:

1. Combine all of the ingredients in a blender.
2. Process until you get a smooth and creamy texture.
3. Bottoms up!

Brain-friendly Smoothie

Ingredients:

- 12 oz. apple juice, organic
- 2 tsp. raw wild honey
- ¾ cup peaches, ripe
- ¾ banana, sliced (without the peeling)
- 2 tsp. flaxseed oil
- 1 tbsp. vanilla-flavored yogurt
- 6 pcs. ice cubes

Directions:

1. Mix all of the ingredients together in a blender.
2. Process until you achieve a smooth and creamy texture.
3. Drink up for a sharper brain. You can turn this into a quick snack or breakfast by drinking it right in the kitchen or by taking it to go!

Coco-Curry Sweet Potato Roast

Ingredients:

- 2 big sweet potatoes
- 2 tbsp. olive oil, extra virgin
- 1 tbsp. curry powder
- 1 tsp. sea salt

Directions:

1. Wash and scrub the sweet potatoes. Dry them. Make sure that you slice off the bruised areas. Then, chop them up into chunks that are about 2 inches in size.
2. Meanwhile, warm up the oven to 415 F.
3. Combine the sweet potato slices and the olive oil in a bowl.
4. Add the curry powder and the salt. Mix well and make sure that the sweet potatoes are completely coated.
5. Arrange the sweet potatoes in a big baking pan. Spread them out evenly. Then, position the pan in the middle rack of your pre-heated oven.
6. Bake for approximately 45 minutes. Make sure that you flip the sweet

potatoes every 15 minutes so they won't end up burnt.

7. This dish is good for two persons when prepared as a light meal or a snack. If you're going to turn this into a side dish, it can serve up to four persons.

Cinnamon-Broc Coleslaw

Ingredients:

- 12 oz. broccoli, shredded
- 2.25 oz. walnuts
- 3 oz. olive oil
- 3 oz. fresh orange juice
- 2 tsp. ground cinnamon
- 4.5 oz. dried cranberries
- 1 tsp. ground ginger
- 4.5 oz. raisins

Directions:

1. In a small bowl, combine the olive oil with the orange juice.
2. Add the cinnamon powder and the ginger powder. Mix well.
3. In a salad bowl, mix the rest of the ingredients together.
4. Pour the vinaigrette over the coleslaw mix and toss well.
5. Cover the salad bowl with cling wrap and place it in the fridge. Keep it there for half an hour.
6. Enjoy your snack! You can also use this as a side dish for a larger meal. Check

out the next chapter for delightful MIND recipes fit for lunch and dinner.

Chapter 4

Big Meals to Fuel Your Brain

Pigeon Peas and Veggies

Not only are pigeon peas uniquely flavorful, they're also rich in protein and fiber!

Ingredients:

- 15 oz. pigeon peas
- 15 oz. ripe tomatoes, cut into chunks
- A cupful of fresh corn kernels
- 1 green bell pepper, sliced thinly
- 1 red bell pepper, sliced thinly
- 1 tbsp. olive oil, extra virgin
- 1 small-sized onion, sliced thinly
- sea salt
- black pepper, freshly ground
- some cayenne pepper (optional)

Directions:

1. Drain the pigeon peas.
2. Adjust the stove's setting to mid-high.

3. In a medium-sized pan, heat the olive oil.
4. Add the onions and the bell peppers and sauté for about 10 minutes.
5. Next, throw in the peas. Add the tomatoes as well.
6. Continue cooking in medium heat for 15 more minutes.
7. Afterwards, put the corn in the pan and cook for a couple of minutes more.
8. Add salt and pepper for seasoning. You may also add cayenne if you wish.
9. For a heavier meal, you can use this recipe as rice toppings.
10. The proportions in this recipe are good for four persons. Following the guidelines of the Mediterranean diet, it's highly recommended that you share this meal with wonderful people that provide stimulating company.

Coco-Cashew Chicken

Ingredients:

- ½ kg organic chicken breasts, boneless
- 96 g cashews, unsalted
- 14 oz. unsweetened coconut milk
- 2 tbsp. organic tomato paste
- ½ tsp. Worcestershire sauce
- 1 big onion, sliced into small cubes
- 1 tsp. turmeric powder
- 1 tbsp. garlic, finely chopped
- 2 tsp. soy sauce, low-sodium brand
- ½ tsp. ground garlic
- black pepper, freshly ground
- ½ tsp. ground onion
- a pinch of sea salt

Directions:

1. Slice the chicken into cubes.
2. Then, place it inside a slow cooker.
3. Add the onions.

4. Add a tiny bit of salt and some pepper as seasoning.
5. Next, throw the rest of the ingredients together in a blender. Process until you create a mixture with a smooth consistency.
6. Pour the mixture all over the chicken cubes.
7. Adjust the slow cooker's setting to low and then cook for about 7 hours.
8. Afterwards, adjust the slow cooker's setting to high. Continue cooking for four more hours.

Note: For a heavier meal, you can use this recipe to make toppings for your preferred grain meal.

Bean and Eggplant Stew

Ingredients:

- 3 eggplants
- 17 oz. fava beans
- 2 oz. precooked anchovies
- 4 big tomatoes, chopped
- 1 medium-sized zucchini sliced
- 1 garlic clove, finely chopped
- 2 tbsp. olive oil, extra virgin
- 2 tsp. organic tomato paste
- a dozen kalamata olives
- a dozen capers
- ½ tsp. marjoram
- sea salt
- ½ tsp. coriander
- black pepper, freshly ground

Directions:

1. Cut up the eggplants to half-inch cubes. Chop up the olives and the capers.
2. Meanwhile, preheat the oven to 425 F.

3. Get a glass baking pan and use a tablespoonful of the olive oil to coat the bottom.
4. Arrange the tomatoes in one layer at the bottom of the baking pan.
5. Place the baking dish in the oven and cook the tomatoes for half an hour. Flip them over. Then, bake for another half an hour.
6. In a large pan, heat the extra tablespoonful of olive oil.
7. Adjust the stove's setting to medium.
8. Sauté the eggplant for about 15 minutes.
9. Next, throw the rest of the ingredients into the pan.
10. Cover the pan and then lower the heat. Leave to cook for about 43 to 46 minutes.
11. When the tomatoes are done, cut them into pieces and toss them into the pan.
12. Replace the lid of the skillet and cook for an extra 40 minutes more. Stir occasionally.
13. The proportions in this recipe can make a meal that's enough for four persons. You can eat this dish alone or serve it over rice if you need something a little heavier.

Pumpkin Patties

Ingredients:

- 15 oz. pureed pumpkin
- 15 oz. kidney beans
- 1 tsp. capers, chopped
- 1 big egg, organic
- 2 tbsp. spring onions, chopped
- 50 g breadcrumbs
- 1 tbsp. cilantro
- 1 tbsp. olive oil
- 2 tsp. lime juice
- 68 g flour
- natural sea salt
- freshly ground black pepper

Directions:

1. Pour the pumpkin puree into a food processor. Throw in the beans and the capers as well. Add the spring onion, the lime juice, and the cilantro. Add half a teaspoonful of sea salt.
2. Process until completely mixed.

3. Next, break the egg and add it into the mixture. This is to be followed by the breadcrumbs.

4. Mix well, making sure that you spread the egg and the crumbs evenly.

5. Add salt and black pepper for seasoning.

6. Afterwards, create patties by shaping the mixture into even-sized balls and flattening them with your palms.

7. Sprinkle flour over a clean, flat work area. Slap each side of each patty on the flour so both sides are covered.

8. Adjust the stove's setting to medium-high.

9. Heat the olive oil in a big pan.

10. Cook the patties. Three minutes on each side should suffice. You'll know they're ready when they yield a nice golden brown color.

11. This recipe makes 6 delicious and nutritious patties.

Quinoa Curry

Ingredients:

- 12 oz. of the Memory Broth (see chapter 2 for recipe)
- 96 g quinoa, rinsed
- 32 g basil leaves, chopped
- 1 tsp. curry powder
- 32 g silvered almonds, toasted
- 6 scallions, chopped
- 2 tbsp. olive oil, extra virgin
- 32 g dried cherries, cut into smaller pieces
- 1 tsp. fresh ginger, finely chopped
- a pinch of natural sea salt
- 2 ½ tbsp. lemon juice
- a pinch of black pepper, freshly ground

Directions:

1. Adjust the stove's setting to high.
2. Pour the Memory Broth into a medium-sized saucepan. Boil.

3. Once it starts boiling, reduce the stove's setting to medium-low.

4. Add the quinoa. Also throw in the minced ginger and the curry powder.

5. Replace the lid of the saucepan and leave to simmer for approximately 20 minutes.

6. Next, place the quinoa on a lined baking dish. Make sure that you spread it evenly.

7. Leave to cool down to room temperature.

8. Then, transfer the cooled quinoa into a bowl.

9. Throw in the almonds and the cherries. Also add the scallions and the basil.

10. Dust off with some pepper and salt. Mix well.

11. Drizzle the lemon juice all over the quinoa. Follow this up with the olive oil. Mix well.

12. Chill before serving.

13. This recipe is for sharing. The proportions here can nourish up to four people.

Mouth-watering Baked Bohemian Squash Recipe

Ingredients:

- 2 medium-sized Bohemian squash

Directions:

1. First, warm up the oven to 375 F.
2. Meanwhile, cut the squash into halves.
3. Prepare a large baking pan and pour in approximately ¼ inch of water.
4. Arrange the squash in the baking pan with the sliced side facing downward.
5. Place the dish in the oven and cook for between 43-46 minutes.
6. Then, flip the squash over and continue baking for 18-22 minutes more. You'll know it's ready when the flesh is all soft.
7. That's it! Enjoy your simple, filling, and nutrition-packed meal!
8. The proportions in this recipe are good for 4 persons.

Roasted Chicken with Sage

Like rosemary, sage is another popular herb which sharpens the memory. Meanwhile, the flavonoids contained in thyme helps increase the brain's antioxidant capacity while its vitamin B6 content positively affects the brain's neurotransmitters to aid in stress reduction.

Ingredients:

- 1.3 kg chicken drumsticks, organic (keep the skin on)
- 1 tbsp. olive oil
- 1 tsp. thyme
- 11 pcs fresh sage

Directions:

1. Wash the sage and dry it.
2. Carefully lift the skin away from the flesh of the chicken and fill each drumstick with equal amounts of dried sage leaves. Make sure that the herb covers about one half of the meat.
3. Heat up the oven to 375 F.
4. Meanwhile, spread olive oil at the bottom of a glass baking pan.

5. Roll the marinated drumsticks in the pan so that each piece is completely coated with oil.

6. Arrange the drumsticks in the baking dish with the skin side down.

7. Use half a teaspoonful of the thyme to sprinkle on top of the meat.

8. Place the glass dish in the oven and bake for about 43-26 minutes.

9. After this, flip the meat over. Sprinkle with the remaining half a teaspoonful of thyme. Continue baking for another 19-21 minutes. You'll know it's ready if the skin is crispy and shows a nice golden hue.

10. You can eat this dish alone or serve it with some potatoes, green beans, or rice for a heavier meal.

11. This recipe can serve up to five.

Chickpeas Stew

Ingredients:

- 30 oz. chickpeas
- 6 big Swiss chard leaves, sliced into fine pieces
- 2 ½ tbsp. olive oil, extra virgin
- 8 oz. fresh tomatoes, cut into cubes
- 1 tbsp. parsley, minced
- 1 medium-sized onion, sliced
- 1 stalk of celery, minced
- 1 clove of garlic, pressed
- a teaspoonful of lemon juice
- grated parmesan (optional)

Directions:

1. In a big pot, immerse the chickpeas in water that's about an inch deep. Partially cover the pot with the lid while allowing it to simmer for about 60 minutes.
2. Meanwhile, adjust the stove's setting to medium.
3. Heat the olive oil. Sauté the onions and the garlic. Stir fry the Swiss chards, the

celery, and the parsley. Do this for half an hour.

4. Drain the chickpeas.
5. Next, throw the peas into the stir-fried mixture.
6. Then, add the tomatoes and the lemon juice.
7. Adjust the stove's setting to low and cook the stew for about 60 minutes more.
8. Use the parmesan cheese as toppings and serve.
9. This recipe is enough to feed 5-6 persons. You can serve it alone or with rice.

Greek-Style Roasted Potatoes

Ingredients:

- 1.3 kg potatoes, chopped into one inch cubes
- 16 oz. vegetable broth
- 2 tbsp. white wine vinegar
- 2.6 oz. olive oil, extra virgin
- 2 tbsp. fresh lemon juice
- 1 ½ tsp. oregano, dehydrated
- fresh parsley, chopped
- 4 cloves garlic, minced
- black pepper, freshly ground
- 1 tsp. kosher salt

Directions:

1. First, warm up the oven to 400 F.
2. Place all of the ingredients save for the fresh herbs and the veggie broth in a big baking pan.
3. Stir the potatoes so that they're fully covered with the olive oil.
4. Pour in the vegetable broth.

5. Place the dish in the oven and bake for approximately 43-46 minutes.

6. Flip the potatoes over. Cook for an extra 25-28 minutes. You'll know they're ready when you pierce the potatoes with a fork and it passes through without resistance.

7. Top with chopped parsley before serving.

8. This recipe can serve up to six.

MIND Japanese-style Soba with Sea Veggies

Ingredients:

- 7 oz. soba noodles
- 10 oz. shitake mushrooms, fresh, sliced
- a couple of sheets of nori, sliced into strips
- 2 oz. water
- 1 ½ medium-sized carrots, cut into strips
- 2 tsp. olive oil
- 1 tbsp. vinegar
- 2 tsp. low-sodium soy sauce

Directions:

1. Adjust the stove's setting to medium heat.
2. Heat the olive oil in a wok and then add the julienned carrots.
3. After sautéing, pour in the water. Follow this up with the vinegar.
4. Cook the carrots until all the liquid has dried up.

5. Throw in the mushrooms and the strips of nori.
6. Continue cooking for three more minutes with occasional stirring.
7. Pour in the soy sauce and stir.
8. Cook the soba noodles.
9. Top the noodles with the stir-fried veggies.
10. This recipe serves 4.

MIND Pasta Salad

Ingredients:

- 450 g fusilli, whole wheat
- 8 big tomatoes, sun-dried
- 1 big ripe tomato, cut into cubes
- 96 g kalamata olives, chopped
- half a red pepper, cut into strips
- half a green pepper, cut into strips
- 2 cloves of garlic, pressed
- 5.5 oz. olive oil, extra virgin
- 2 oz. red wine vinegar
- black pepper, freshly ground
- ½ tsp. kosher salt

Directions:

1. Cook the fusilli, drain, and then use the olive oil to coat the pasta completely. Leave to cool to room temperature.
2. In a separate bowl, place the sun-dried tomatoes. Add two volumes of red wine vinegar and water. Leave for about 7 minutes.

3. Once the tomatoes are tender, cut them into small pieces that are about a quarter of an inch in size.

4. Add the tomatoes to the fusilli. Also add the rest of the ingredients to the pasta bowl. Mix well.

5. Scoop the pasta into serving dishes. Use fresh parsley for garnishing.

6. This can feed up to 7 individuals. Serve cold. For a fuller, more nutritious meal, eat this with some stir-fried zucchini.

Baked Salmon and Sweet Potatoes with Kale

Ingredients:

- 450 g salmon filet
- 1 medium-sized sweet potato
- 3 1/2 tbsp. olive oil
- a bundle of fresh kale
- 12 pcs. cherry tomatoes
- 1 medium-sized orange
- 1 medium-sized lemon
- 1 medium-sized grapefruit
- 1 ½ tsp. sea salt
- 2 tsp. black pepper, freshly ground

Directions:

1. Heat up the oven to 400 F.
2. Prepare a 13 x 9 sized baking dish.
3. Grate the sweet potatoes into very thin shreds.
4. Coat them with a tablespoonful of olive oil. Also squeeze a tablespoonful of fresh orange juice and half a teaspoonful of fresh orange zest. Add one teaspoonful

of freshly ground black pepper and half a teaspoonful of natural sea salt.

5. Arrange half of the sweet potatoes on the right side of the baking pan.

6. Slice the kale into pieces after rinsing the leaves. Coat with a tablespoonful of olive oil, a tablespoonful of grapefruit juice and half a teaspoonful of grapefruit zest. Also add half a teaspoonful each of salt and black pepper. Arrange the kale on the left side of the baking pan.

7. Slice the salmon filet into half. Coat with the remaining olive oil. Slather with a tablespoonful of lemon juice and add half a teaspoonful of lemon zest. Also add the remaining sea salt and pepper.

8. Arrange the salmon filets betwixt the kale and the sweet potatoes. Make sure that the skin side is facing downward.

9. Drizzle with some more olive oil and top with a slice of lemon.

10. Arrange the cherry tomatoes on top of the salmon filets.

11. Place in the oven and cook for about 23-26 minutes.

Thai-style Wheat Salad

Ingredients:

- 128 g wheat berries
- 28 oz. water
- 4.5 oz. tomatoes, chopped
- 5 tbsp. olive oil, extra virgin
- 2 tsp. curry powder
- 1 scallion, chopped
- juice from 1 lime
- 1 tbsp. cilantro, fresh, sliced
- black pepper, freshly ground
- sea salt
- unsalted peanuts (for toppings)

Directions:

1. In a big saucepan, place the wheat berries. Then pour in the water. Boil.
2. Once it's boiling, replace the lid of the saucepan and lower the heat.
3. Leave to simmer for 46-60 minutes.
4. Next, drain the wheat berries while rinsing them in cool water.

5. In a small bowl, mix the olive oil with the lime juice.

6. Throw in the curry powder and add some salt. Sprinkle with pepper. Whisk well until thoroughly combined.

7. In a bigger bowl, transfer the wheat berries. Then, add the tomatoes, the cilantro, and the scallions.

8. Drizzle the dressing all over the salad. Toss well until all the wheat berries are fully coated.

9. Top with unsalted peanuts. Serve at once after preparing.

Salmon Beet Salad

Ingredients:

For the salad:

- 170 g salmon flakes, precooked
- 64 g beets, cooked
- 3 cupsful of romaine lettuce
- 12 pcs. pistachios, chopped
- a quarter of a medium-sized avocado, cut into cubes
- 1 big-sized orange, coarsely chopped
- 1 red onion, finely chopped

For the vinaigrette:

- 2 tbsp. white wine vinegar
- 1 tbsp. olive oil, extra virgin
- ½ tsp. Dijon mustard
- 2 tbsp. orange juice, freshly squeezed
- ½ tsp., orange zest
- freshly ground black pepper
- ¼ tsp. chili powder
- a pinch of kosher salt

Directions:

1. Mix all of the ingredients for the vinaigrette in a bowl. Whisk well until you arrive at a smooth texture.
2. In a salad bowl, mix the salmon and the romaine lettuce. Add the avocado and the orange slices and toss again.
3. Add the beets and the onions. Toss.
4. Pour the dressing over the bed of romaine and toss again.
5. Use the pistachio nuts as toppings before digging in.

Chicken Piccata

Ingredients:

- 2 pcs. organic chicken breasts, butterflied
- 4 oz. chicken broth, reduced sodium
- 5 oz. portabella mushrooms, chopped
- 2.6 oz. fresh lemon juice
- 45 g almond flour
- 32 g capers
- 2.6 oz. parsley, fresh, sliced
- 6 tbsp. virgin coconut oil
- 5 tbsp. olive oil, extra virgin
- sea salt
- freshly ground black pepper

Directions:

1. Use desired amount of pepper and just a little bit of salt to season the chicken meat.
2. Place the almond flour in a big bowl and roll the meat in the flour until both sides are fully covered. Shake off any extra flour.
3. Adjust the stove's setting to medium high.

4. Heat two tablespoonsful of coconut oil and three tablespoonsful olive oil together in a skillet.
5. As the oil begins to sizzle, put two pieces of chicken breast in the pan and cook each side for about three minutes each. Makes sure that both sides are nice and brown.
6. Place the meat in a serving plate.
7. Next, heat another two tablespoonsful each of coconut oil and olive oil.
8. Cook the remaining chicken meat just like the first two.
9. This time, throw in the mushrooms. Stir fry for 4-6 minutes. Decide whether you need to add some more olive oil or coconut oil.
10. Switch off the stove and transfer the chicken to the serving plate.
11. In the same skillet, pour in the chicken stock. Add the lemon juice. Throw in the capers. Leave to boil.
12. Meanwhile, scrape off the brown morsels from the pan for some added

flavor. Season as desired but don't add any more salt.

13. Afterwards, take all the chicken back into the skillet. Cook for an additional 4-6 minutes.
14. Transfer the cooked chicken breasts back to the serving plate.
15. Drizzle the sauce with the rest of the coconut oil. Whisk briskly.
16. Then, pour the sauce all over the chicken breasts.
17. Use the fresh parsley for garnishing.
18. Eat heartily with friendly company.

Tex Mex Chops

Ingredients:

- 12 oz. sirloin chops, boneless
- 2 tsp. olive oil
- 4 oz. green chili peppers, diced
- 9 oz. tomatoes, cubed
- ½ tsp. zero sodium chipotle seasoning

Directions:

1. Adjust the stove's setting to medium-high.
2. Grease a non-stick skillet with the olive oil.
3. Put the chops in the pan. Brown both sides for a couple of minutes each.
4. Next, throw in the chilies and the tomatoes. Add the chipotle seasoning. Mix thoroughly.
5. Replace the lid of the skillet and adjust the stove's setting to low.
6. Cook for approximately 9-12 minutes.
7. Enjoy eating this hearty and succulent meal with people who matter to you!

Chapter 5

Sweet and MIND-ful Treats

MIND Pineapple Smoothie

Ingredients:

- 4 oz. pineapple chunks
- 6 oz. water
- a couple of cupsful of kale, stem removed and leaves chopped to small pieces
- 1 medium-sized apple, core removed
- 1 medium-sized pear, core-removed

Directions:

1. Throw all of the ingredients together in a blender.
2. Pulse until you get a smooth drink.
3. Pour into a tall glass and serve immediately.

Memory-boosting Topical Fusion

Ingredients:

- 8 oz. papaya
- a couple of cupsful of baby spinach
- 1 medium-sized apple, core removed
- 6 oz. almond milk, unsweetened

Directions:

1. Combine all of the ingredients in a blender.
2. Process until smooth.
3. Enjoy your sweet and healthy treat!

Healthy Rosemary and Blueberry Ice Cream

Rosemary is an herb which is known to improve the memory. Just the scent of it can help boost recall by 75%!

Ingredients:

- 8 oz. blueberries
- 1 tsp. fresh rosemary, finely chopped
- 2 yolks from organic eggs
- 14 oz. coconut milk
- 2 tbsp. raw wild honey
- a teaspoonful of lemon juice

Directions:

1. In a food processor, mix the coconut milk and the blueberries. Add the honey and the lemon juice. Throw in the rosemary.
2. Process until all the ingredients are completely blended.
3. Transfer the mixture into a pot.
4. Adjust the stove's setting to medium.
5. Add the egg yolks into the mixture.

6. Bring the mixture to a low boil with continuous and brisk stirring.
7. As the mixture starts to boil, switch off the stove and leave it to cool at room temperature.
8. Afterwards, pour the mixture into a bowl. Cover the bowl with cling wrap.
9. Place the bowl in the fridge and leave overnight.
10. The following day, introduce the blend into an ice cream maker.
11. Then, spoon the ice cream into serving bowls.
12. Serve this merry treat to guests.
13. The proportions in this recipe makes one pint of ice cream. You can keep the rest in the freezer.

Note: Don't own an ice cream maker? No worries. Just place the mixture in a bread pan and keep it in the freezer. After it's frozen, thaw for about 15 minutes so you can spoon this memory-boosting cold treat easily into serving cups.

Brain-enhancing Blueberry Crumble

Ingredients:

- 2 cupsful of blueberries
- 4.8 oz. almond meal
- 32 g macadamia, chopped
- 2 oz. virgin coconut oil, melted
- ¼ tsp. cinnamon
- 3 tbsp. lemon juice
- a couple of pinches of natural sea salt

Directions:

1. First, warm up the oven to 375 F.
2. Arrange the berries in a 9 x 9 sized baking tin.
3. Pour 1 1/2 tbsp. of lemon juice all over the blueberries. Toss a bit to ensure that all berries are coated with lemon extract.
4. Place the almond meal in a bowl. Add the coconut oil and throw in the chopped macadamia nuts.
5. Pour the rest of the lemon juice into the bowl.

6. Sprinkle with salt and cinnamon. Mix well.
7. Once the nut spread is ready, slather it all over the berries.
8. Bake in the oven for half an hour to 39 minutes. The top of the blueberry crumble should have a nice golden brown hue.

MIND Walnut Fudge

Ingredients:

- 8 oz. coconut oil
- 57 g almond butter, organic
- 34 g raw cacao, unsweetened
- 32 g walnuts, chopped
- 3 oz. maple syrup, organic
- 1 tsp. vanilla bean extract

Directions:

1. Place all of the above ingredients in a bowl and mix thoroughly.
2. Spread the mixture uniformly in a 5 x 9 sized glass baking dish.
3. Stick the baking dish in the freezer and leave it there for 30 minutes or more.
4. This recipe serves 8 so feel free to share this heavenly treat.
5. Indulge!

Note: Always chill the fudge before serving because this dessert has a tendency to melt when kept in room temperature.

MIND Diet Chocolate Cookie Recipe

Ingredients:

- 8 oz. avocado slices, ripe
- 1 egg. organic
- 1 large banana, sliced
- 68 g raw cocoa, unsweetened
- ½ tsp. baking soda
- 1 tbsp. raw wild honey
- Semisweet chocolate chips (optional)

Directions:

1. First, heat up the oven to 350 F.
2. In a mixing bowl, place the avocado slices and the banana slices. Mash them together.
3. Then, pour in the raw wild honey and mix well.
4. Transfer the batter into a food processor.
5. Break in the egg. Add the cocoa and the baking powder.
6. Pulse until completely blended.

7. Prepare a baking sheet by lining it with parchment paper.
8. If you're using chocolate chips for this recipe, now is the time to stir them in.
9. Arrange spoonsful of the dough on the baking dish while making sure that they're evenly spaced.
10. Place the baking dish in the oven and bake for about 9 minutes.
11. Feel free to go crazy with this dessert. Your brain and your body will thank you for it!

Just Peachy MIND-ful Blueberry Smoothie

Ingredients:

- 6 oz. blueberries
- 5 oz. water
- a couple of medium-sized peaches, pits removed
- a couple of leaves of collard greens
- 1 celery stalk

Directions:

1. Combine all of the ingredients in a blender.
2. Pulse until you obtain a perfectly smooth texture.
3. Gulp down for a fit body and a sharp mind!

MIND Diet Quick Yogurt Dessert

Ingredients:

- 17g ml zero fat plain yogurt
- 2 tbsp. almonds, chopped
- ½ tsp. raw wild honey
- 1 tbsp. grated coconut, unsweetened
- 6 oz. fresh raspberries

Directions:

1. In a cup, combine the raw wild honey and the yogurt. Mix well.
2. Add the coconut strips and the chopped almonds. Stir with a teaspoon.
3. Add the raspberries as toppings.
4. Pamper your taste buds with this delightful dessert while knowing that it's oh-so-good for your mind and your body too!

Conclusion

Thank you again for buying this book!

I hope this book was able to help you learn how to prepare delightful and nourishing meals that will aid in decreasing your chances of developing Alzheimer's disease in the future while keeping your mind and your body fit in the present.

The next step is to start raiding your pantry and get rid of the unhealthy ingredients that you no longer need. Switch to the MIND diet and embrace the MIND lifestyle by pairing your diet with regular exercise.

As repeatedly emphasized throughout this book, make it a habit to share meals with loved ones and with guests that provide good and stimulating company. Regular social activity and an effective support system also helps lower the risks of developing Alzheimer's.

Thank you and good luck!

Made in the USA
Middletown, DE
09 March 2017